DIABETES

MENU FOR CARING FOR A DIABETIC PATIENCE

DR. LEROY MCCARTHY

Contents

CHAPTER ONE

INTRODUCTION

Diabetes is a not unusual condition that influences human beings of every age. There are numerous sorts of diabetes. Type 2 is the most commonplace. A mixture of treatment techniques can help you manage the state of affairs to stay a healthful lifestyles and prevent headaches.

Diabetes is a situation that takes area while your blood sugar (glucose) is just too excessive. It develops while your pancreas doesn't make enough insulin or any the least bit, or when your frame isn't responding to the outcomes of insulin well. Diabetes impacts human beings of all ages. Most styles of diabetes are persistent (lifelong), and all bureaucracy are capability with drugs and/or lifestyle adjustments.

Glucose (sugar) particularly comes from carbohydrates in your food and drink. It's your frame's move-to deliver of strength. Your blood incorporates glucose to all your frame's cells to apply for strength.

Whilst glucose is to your bloodstream, it goals assist — a "key" — to attain its very last holiday spot. This key's insulin (a hormone). In case your pancreas isn't making enough insulin or your body isn't using it well, glucose builds up to your bloodstream, inflicting immoderate blood sugar (hyperglycemia).

Through the years, having constantly high

blood glucose can purpose fitness problems, in conjunction with heart ailment, nerve harm and eye problems.

The technical call for diabetes is diabetes mellitus. Every other state of affairs shares the term "diabetes" — diabetes insipidus — however they're exceptional. They percentage the name "diabetes" due to the reality they every reason extended thirst and common urination. Diabetes insipidus is lots rarer than diabetes mellitus.

Diabetes mellitus refers to a collection of sicknesses which have an impact on how the body makes use of blood sugar (glucose). Glucose is an critical source of electricity for the cells that make up the muscular tissues and tissues. It's also the mind's primary supply of gasoline.

The primary purpose of diabetes varies by way of type. However regardless of what form of diabetes you've got, it is able to purpose extra sugar in the blood. Too much sugar in the blood can purpose intense health issues.

Chronic diabetes situations consist of type 1 diabetes and type 2 diabetes. Likely reversible diabetes situations include prediabetes and gestational diabetes. Prediabetes occurs at the same time as blood sugar ranges are higher than everyday. But the blood sugar levels are not excessive enough to be called diabetes. And prediabetes can lead to diabetes except steps are taken to prevent it. Gestational diabetes takes place at some point of being pregnant. But it may depart after the toddler is born.

Diabetes, additionally called diabetes mellitus, is a circumstance that influences insulin, a hormone that breaks down sugars inside the food you consume and converts them into glucose to gasoline the body.

Diabetes takes place whilst your body does no longer system meals as power nicely. Insulin is a crucial hormone that receives glucose (sugar that is used as power) to the cells on your frame. When you have diabetes, your body both doesn't reply to insulin or doesn't produce insulin the least bit. This motives sugars to build up to your blood, which places you vulnerable to risky headaches.

What are the styles of diabetes?

There are various sorts of diabetes. The maximum commonplace bureaucracy embody:

Type 2 diabetes: With this kind, your body doesn't make sufficient insulin and/or your body's cells don't respond usually to the insulin (insulin resistance). That is the maximum common form of diabetes. It especially affects adults, however kids will have it as nicely.

Prediabetes: This kind is the level in advance than kind 2 diabetes. Your blood glucose tiers are better than everyday but not high sufficient to be formally identified with type

2 diabetes.

Kind 1 diabetes: This kind is an autoimmune disease in which your immune system attacks and destroys insulin-producing cells on your pancreas for unknown reasons. Up to ten% of people who've diabetes have kind 1. It's usually recognized in kids and young adults, but it is able to amplify at any age.

Gestational diabetes: This type develops in a few people at some point of pregnancy. Gestational diabetes generally is going away after pregnancy. But, when you have gestational diabetes, you're at a better threat of growing kind 2 diabetes later in lifestyles.

Exceptional kinds of diabetes include:

Type 3c diabetes: This shape of diabetes takes place whilst your pancreas memories damage (other than autoimmune harm), which impacts its potential to offer insulin. Pancreatitis, pancreatic most cancers, cystic fibrosis and hemochromatosis can all result in pancreas damage that reasons diabetes. Having your pancreas eliminated (pancreatectomy) also outcomes in kind 3c.

Latent autoimmune diabetes in adults (LADA): Like type 1 diabetes, LADA additionally results from an autoimmune reaction, however it develops plenty greater slowly than kind 1. People identified with LADA are usually over the age of 30.

Adulthood-onset diabetes of the younger (MODY): MODY, additionally referred to as monogenic diabetes, takes region due to an inherited genetic mutation that influences how your frame makes and uses insulin. There are presently over 10 unique varieties of MODY. It affects as plenty as 5% of humans with diabetes and commonly runs in households.

Neonatal diabetes: that may be a uncommon form of diabetes that takes area within the first six months of lifestyles. It's additionally a form of monogenic diabetes. Approximately 50% of infants with neonatal diabetes have the lifelong shape called everlasting neonatal diabetes mellitus. For the alternative 1/2, the situation disappears within a few months from onset, but it is able to come again later in lifestyles. That is known as brief neonatal diabetes mellitus.

Brittle diabetes: Brittle diabetes is a shape of kind 1 diabetes that's marked with the useful resource of frequent and immoderate episodes of excessive and coffee blood sugar stages. This instability frequently ends in hospitalization. In uncommon instances, a pancreas transplant may be essential to completely deal with brittle diabetes.

Signs and symptoms

Diabetes symptoms depend on how excessive your blood sugar is. A few human beings, in particular in the occasion that they've prediabetes, gestational diabetes or kind 2 diabetes, may not have signs and symptoms. In kind 1 diabetes, signs and signs and symptoms will be predisposed to return on speedy and be extra severe.

Feeling greater thirsty than standard.

Urinating frequently.

Dropping weight without attempting.

Presence of ketones in the urine. Ketones are a byproduct of the breakdown of muscle and fats that occurs while there may be no longer enough available insulin.

Feeling tired and susceptible.

Feeling irritable or having distinctive temper adjustments.

Having blurry imaginative and prescient.

Having gradual-recuperation sores.

Getting masses of infections, which include gum, pores and pores and skin and vaginal infections.

Kind 1 diabetes can begin at any age. However it frequently starts offevolved inside the course of youth or youngster years. Type 2 diabetes, the more common type, can growth at any age. Type 2 diabetes is more common in humans older than forty. But type 2 diabetes in youngsters is growing.

CHAPTER TWO

Diabetes prognosis

A medical doctor can diagnose diabetes with one or more of the following blood checks:

Random blood sugar check: Taken any time, no matter how currently you have eaten.

A1C test: Assesses blood sugar degrees over severa months.

Fasting blood sugar check: Measures blood sugar ranges after you haven't eaten in a unmarried day.

Glucose tolerance check: Takes blood levels over the direction of several hours to reveal how short your body metabolizes the glucose in a unique liquid you drink.

Diabetes treatment

Remedy for diabetes relies upon on its kind and severity, and may embody:

Common blood glucose checking to expose blood glucose degrees

Life-style modifications, including weight loss plan and workout

Oral remedy

Each day insulin injections

Everyday bodily checks are vital for humans with any shape of diabetes to reveal and deal with any bobbing up headaches, at the side of eye problems, kidney sickness, cardiovascular disease and neuropathy (harm to the nerves).

What are the complications of diabetes?

Diabetes can bring about acute (sudden and excessive) and lengthy-time period headaches — especially due to excessive or prolonged excessive blood sugar stages.

Acute diabetes headaches

Acute diabetes headaches that can be lifestyles-threatening encompass:

Hyperosmolar hyperglycemic kingdom (HHS): This complication mainly influences human beings with kind 2 diabetes. It occurs when your blood sugar degrees are very high (over 600 milligrams consistent with deciliter or mg/dL) for an prolonged period, main to excessive dehydration and confusion. It calls for immediate scientific remedy.

Diabetes-associated ketoacidosis (DKA): This problem in particular influences humans with kind 1 diabetes or undiagnosed T1D. It takes place when your frame doesn't have sufficient insulin. In case your body doesn't have insulin, it may't use glucose for energy, so it breaks down fats instead. This system in the long run releases substances referred to as ketones, which turn your blood acidic. This motives labored respiration, vomiting and lack of interest. DKA requires straight away clinical remedy.

Extreme low blood sugar (hypoglycemia): Hypoglycemia takes place at the same time as your blood sugar diploma drops beneath the range that's healthy for you. Extreme hypoglycemia may be very low blood sugar. It specifically influences humans with diabetes who use insulin. Signs and symptoms include blurred or double vision, clumsiness, disorientation and seizures. It calls for treatment with emergency glucagon and/or scientific intervention.

Lengthy-time period diabetes complications

Blood glucose stages that stay excessive for too lengthy can damage your frame's tissues and organs. That is particularly due to harm in your blood vessels and nerves, which assist your frame's tissues.

Cardiovascular (coronary coronary heart and blood vessel) issues are the maximum not unusual sort of long-term diabetes issue. They consist of:

Coronary artery disease.

Coronary coronary heart assault.

Stroke.

Atherosclerosis.

One of a kind diabetes complications include:

Nerve damage (neuropathy), that can reason numbness, tingling and/or pain.

Nephropathy, that may cause kidney failure or the want for dialysis or transplant.

Retinopathy, that may reason blindness.

Diabetes-related foot conditions.

Pores and skin infections.

Amputations.

Sexual disease because of nerve and blood vessel damage, including erectile ailment or vaginal dryness.

Gastroparesis.

Being attentive to loss.

Oral health problems, which include gum (periodontal) disease.

Residing with diabetes can also have an impact to your highbrow fitness. People with diabetes are to 3 times more likely to have despair than human beings with out diabetes.

Prevention

Kind 1 diabetes cannot be prevented. But the healthful manner of existence options that help treat prediabetes, kind 2 diabetes and gestational diabetes also can help save you them:

Eat healthy components. Choose components decrease in fat and energy and better in fiber. Attention on culmination, veggies and whole grains. Eat a spread to hold from feeling bored.

Get more bodily hobby. Try to get approximately 30 minutes of moderate cardio activity on most days of the week. Or intention to get at least a hundred and fifty mins of moderate cardio interest per week. For example, take a brisk every day stroll. If you can't healthy in an extended exercising, damage it up into smaller lessons in some unspecified time in the future of the day.

Lose more pounds. If you're obese, losing even 7% of your body weight can lower the danger of diabetes. For instance, if you weigh two hundred kilos (ninety.7 kilograms), losing 14 pounds (6.Four kilograms) can decrease the danger of diabetes.

However do not try to lose weight all through pregnancy. Speak to your organisation about how a good buy weight is healthful with a view to gain during pregnancy.

To maintain your weight in a wholesome variety, paintings on long-time period modifications to your consuming and exercising behavior. Bear in mind the benefits of dropping weight, together with a greater wholesome coronary heart, greater electricity and better vanity.

Conclusion

Being recognized with diabetes is a lifestyles-converting occasion, but it doesn't imply you may't stay a satisfied and healthful lifestyles. Coping with diabetes includes consistent care and diligence. At the same time as it'll likely be very overwhelming earlier than the whole thing, over time you'll get a higher keep close on managing the circumstance and being in track together with your frame.

Make sure to peer your healthcare provider(s) frequently. Dealing with diabetes involves a team attempt — you'll want clinical experts, friends and circle of relatives in your aspect. Don't be afraid to acquire out to them if you need assist.

THE END